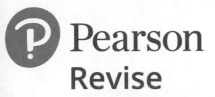

Pearson
Revise

Revise BTEC Tech Award

Sport (2022)

Practice Assessments Plus⁺

Series Consultant: Harry Smith

Author: Sue Hartigan

A note from the publisher

While the publishers have made every attempt to ensure that advice on the qualification and its assessment is accurate, the official specification and associated assessment guidance materials are the only authoritative source of information and should always be referred to for definitive guidance.

This qualification is reviewed on a regular basis and may be updated in the future.

Any such updates that affect the content of this Revision Guide will be outlined at

www.pearsonfe.co.uk/BTECchanges. The eBook version of this Revision Guide will also be updated to reflect the latest guidance as soon as possible.

> **For the full range of Pearson revision titles across KS2, KS3, GCSE, Functional Skills, AS/A Level and BTEC visit:**
> www.pearsonschools.co.uk/revise

Published by Pearson Education Limited, 80 Strand, London, WC2R 0RL.

www.pearsonschoolsandfecolleges.co.uk

Copies of official specifications for all Pearson qualifications may be found on the website: qualifications.pearson.com

Text and illustrations © Pearson Education Ltd 2022

Typeset, produced and illustrated by PDQ Media

Cover illustration © Simple Line/Shutterstock

The right of Sue Hartigan to be identified as author of this work has been asserted by her in accordance with the Copyright, Designs and Patents Act 1988.

First published 2022

25 24

10 9 8 7 6

British Library Cataloguing in Publication Data

A catalogue record for this book is available from the British Library

ISBN 978 1 292 43630 2

Acknowledgements

1: McCardle, W. et al. Extract from Essentials of Exercise Physiology (2nd Edition). © Lippincott Williams and Wilkins, 2000; **17**, **33**, **49**: Davis, B. et al. Extract from Physical Education and the Study of Sport (4th Edition). © Harcourt Publishers, 2000. pp123–124.

Printed in Great Britain by Bell and Bain Ltd, Glasgow

Notes from the publisher

1. While the publishers have made every attempt to ensure that advice on the qualification and its assessment is accurate, the official specification and associated assessment guidance materials are the only authoritative source of information and should always be referred to for definitive guidance. Pearson examiners have not contributed to any sections in this resource relevant to examination papers for which they have responsibility.

2. Pearson has robust editorial processes, including answer and fact checks, to ensure the accuracy of the content in this publication, and every effort is made to ensure this publication is free of errors. We are, however, only human, and occasionally errors do occur. Pearson is not liable for any misunderstandings that arise as a result of errors in this publication, but it is our priority to ensure that the content is accurate. If you spot an error, please do contact us at resourcescorrections@pearson.com so we can make sure it is corrected.

Websites

Pearson Education Limited is not responsible for the content of any external internet sites. It is essential for tutors to preview each website before using it in class so as to ensure that the URL is still accurate, relevant and appropriate. We suggest that tutors bookmark useful websites and consider enabling students to access them through the school/college intranet.

Introduction

This book has been designed to help you to practise the skills you may need for the external assessment of BTEC Tech Award **Sport**, Component 3: Developing Fitness to Improve Other Participants Performance in Sport and Physical Activity

About the practice assessments

The book contains four practice assessments for the component. Unlike your actual assessment, the questions have targeted hints, guidance and support in the margin to help you understand how to tackle them:

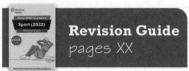 links to relevant pages in the Pearson Revise BTEC Tech Award Sport Revision Guide so you can revise the essential content. This will also help you to understand how the essential content is applied to different contexts when assessed.

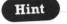 to get you started and remind you of the skills or knowledge you need to apply.

 to help you on how to approach a question, such as making a brief plan.

 to provide content that you need to learn such as a definition or principles related to training, nutrition and psychology.

 to help you avoid common pitfalls.

 to remind you of content related to the question to aid your revision on that topic.

 for use with the final practice assessment to help you become familiar with answering in a given time and ways to think about allocating time for different questions.

There is space for you to write your answers to the questions within this book. However, if you require more space to complete your answers, you may want to use separate paper.

There is also an answer section at the back of the book, so you can check your answers for each practice assessment.

Check the Pearson website

For overarching guidance on the official assessment outcomes and key terms used in your assessment, please refer to the specification on the Pearson website. Check also whether you must have a calculator in your assessment.

The practice questions, support and answers in this book are provided to help you to revise the essential content in the specification, along with ways of applying your skills. Details of your actual assessment may change, so always make sure you are up to date on its format and requirements by asking your tutor or checking the Pearson website for the most up-to-date Sample Assessment Material, Mark Schemes and any past papers.

Contents

A small bit of small print

Pearson publishes Sample Assessment Material and the specification on its website. This is the official content and this book should be used in conjunction with it. The questions have been written to help you test your knowledge and skills. Remember: the real assessment may not look like this.

Practice assessment 1

Answer ALL questions.
Write your answers in the spaces provided.

Some questions must be answered with a cross in a box ☒. If you change your mind about an answer, put a line through the box ☒ and then mark your new answer with a cross ☒.

Raj takes part in the sit and reach test. His sit and reach test score is **11 cm**. **Table 1** shows the normative test data for the sit and reach test.

	Category			
Gender	**Above average**	**Average**	**Below average**	**Very poor**
Male	>14.1	14.0	13.9–9.1	<9
Female	>15.1	15.0	14.9–10.1	<10

Table 1

1 (a) Which **one** of the following is Raj's rating for the sit and reach test?

  ☐ **A** Above average

  ☐ **B** Average

  ☐ **C** Below average

  ☐ **D** Very poor

`1 mark`

(b) Name the component of fitness tested by the sit and reach test.

....

`1 mark`

Raj carries out some pre-test procedures before fitness testing.

(c) Which **one** of the following must be carried out before fitness testing?

  ☐ **A** Calculation of training zones

  ☐ **B** Calibration of equipment

  ☐ **C** Cool down

  ☐ **D** Setting SMART targets

`1 mark`

Revision Guide
page 26

LEARN IT!

The symbol > means greater than. The symbol < means less than. For **Table 1**, a male scoring more than 14.1 (>14.1) rates above average, or less than 9 (<9) rates very poor.

Hint

In a multiple-choice question, you need to read each of the options carefully and discount any that you know are not correct, you can then decide on the right answer.

Prepare

As well as the sit and reach test, make sure you know the calf muscle flexibility test and the shoulder flexibility test. Consider how well each test design allows it to measure the component of fitness and the practicality and validity of these tests for different sports and participants.

Hint

For a **name** question you need to give a brief, precise answer. There is no need to add any explanation.

Hint

In Question 1(c) mark the box clearly with an 'X' so that the examiner is sure which answer you have chosen.

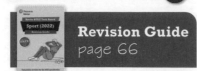

Revision Guide
page 66

LEARN IT!

Sprint hurdling is where athletes run as fast as they can and also jump to clear a number of hurdles as they run.

Hint

If asked to **state**, recall the correct name from the specification. For example, a training method to improve **strength** would be 'free weights'.

Hint

Give valid reasons for each of the selected training methods. For example, if the sport was rowing, which requires strength, a reason for choosing free weights would be that it is easy to target the muscles that require increased strength so they can exert more force on the water to go faster.

LEARN IT!

Personal goals can be remembered by the mnemonic SMARTER:
S – specific
M – measurable
A – achievable
R – realistic
T – time-related
E – exciting
R – recorded

Hint

In Question 1(f) **explain** requires you to correctly identify a reason and then provide further details to give an explanation as to why this is.

Raj is a sprint hurdler. He uses two different training methods to improve his power and speed.

(d) Complete **Table 2** by stating:

    (i) **one** method of training to improve each component of fitness

    (ii) **one** reason why each method of training is suitable for Raj.

Component of fitness	(i) Method of training	(ii) Reason why method of training is suitable
Power	....	....
Speed	....	....

Table 2

`4 marks`

Raj motivates himself to improve his fitness by setting personal goals. A measurable goal is an example of a personal goal.

(e) Name **one** other type of personal goal.

....

....

`1 mark`

Goal setting has a number of benefits.

(f) Explain **one** reason why Raj should set measurable goals.

....

....

....

....

`2 marks`

Total for Question 1 = 10 marks

Table 3 shows Ivan's weekly training plan.

Session number	Warm-up	Main activity	Time spent on main activity
1	Pulse-raiser, joint mobilisation and stretching	Running on a treadmill at a constant pace	30 minutes
2	Pulse-raiser, joint mobilisation and stretching	Fartlek training session in the park	30 minutes
3	Pulse-raiser, joint mobilisation and stretching	Swimming continuous lengths in the pool	30 minutes

Table 3

2 (a) Using the information in **Table 3**

(i) Identify the principle of training Ivan is applying in his training.

....

....

1 mark

(ii) Identify the component of fitness Ivan is working on in his training plan.

....

....

1 mark

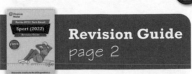

Revision Guide
page 2

Hint

Identify means you need to use the information provided in the question. Ivan uses three different activities in his training plan.

LEARN IT!

Fartlek training involves running at varying speeds and can also be over different terrain. This means the intensity of the training will change during the session.

Hint

In Question 2(a)i the principles of training are the 'rules' followed to make sure that training is effective. For example, progressive overload should be applied by gradually making the training harder. This could be through increasing the time spent exercising, but this isn't happening here as each session is 30 minutes.

Hint

Think about the type of training that lasts 30 minutes.

Hint

You are told that Fartlek training will improve Ivan's aerobic endurance. Training that improves aerobic endurance brings about specific adaptations to the cardiovascular and respiratory systems. Think about these adaptations and how one of these adaptations would help to improve Ivan's aerobic endurance.

LEARN IT!

The Borg (6–20) Rating of Perceived Exertion (RPE) Scale can be used by a performer to estimate exercise intensity or how hard they think/feel they are working.

Hint

When answering the **describe** Question in 2(c) you need to give a clear account of the steps someone would go through to work out their heart rate using the Borg scale. Say what the scale is, what the numbers on the scale mean and then how they are used to work out heart rate.

Hint

In Question 2(d) give the exact meaning of the term.

(b) Explain **one** reason why Ivan's aerobic endurance would improve through regular Fartlek training.

....

....

....

....

2 marks

> In order to improve his fitness Ivan must make sure he is working at the correct intensity.

(c) Describe how Ivan can use the Borg scale to estimate his heart rate during a training session.

....

....

....

....

....

....

3 marks

> Ivan is highly motivated to maintain his training.

(d) Give a definition of the term motivation.

....

....

1 mark

Ivan's motivation comes from himself and from his coach.

(e) Complete **Table 4** by stating:

  (i) the type of motivation given in the description

  (ii) an example of this type of motivation.

Description	(i) Type of motivation	(ii) Example of type of motivation
From within the performer	....	....
From an external source such as a coach	....	....

Table 4

4 marks

Total for Question 2 = 12 marks

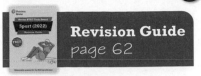

Revision Guide
page 62

LEARN IT!

There are two types of motivation: intrinsic and extrinsic.

Hint

Use your own experience to help you answer this question. Think about your own reasons for participating in physical activity, and what motivates you.

Hint

Double-check your answer to make sure that you have placed your answers in the correct box.

Hint

Even if you are not sure of all the answers, try to complete as much of the table as possible as you will gain marks for any correct answers. For example, if you can only think of one type of motivation, add it to the table even if you have to leave the rest blank.

Revision Guide
pages 1 and 5

Hint

To do well in weightlifting, performers need to lift heavy weights, but they also need to be able to move the heavy weight quickly to lift the weight over their head and then hold it in that position.

Hint

Strength is needed to lift a heavy weight but this isn't given as one of the options. Think about what James needs to move the heavy weight quickly.

LEARN IT!

Power is strength × speed. Power allows us to carry out explosive movements.

Hint

Use of connecting words such as 'because', 'therefore', 'which means that' will help you develop your point in **'explain'** questions.

LEARN IT!

Balance allows the control of the distribution of weight.

James is a weightlifter.

3 (a) Which **one** of the following components of fitness is **most** important to James in his activity?

☐ **A** Agility

☐ **B** Aerobic endurance

☐ **C** Power

☐ **D** Reaction time

1 mark

(b) State **one** reason why James should develop his muscular strength.

....

....

1 mark

James also needs good balance when weightlifting.

(c) Explain **one** reason why James would also need good balance.

....

....

....

....

2 marks

Revision Guide
page 19

James regularly tests his fitness.

(d) Explain **one** reason why James's level of motivation can affect the reliability of his fitness test result.

....

....

....

....

2 marks

James regularly uses fitness tests to test his strength.

(e) Explain **two** reasons for regularly carrying out fitness testing.

1 ....

....

....

....

2 ....

....

....

....

4 marks

Hint

Reliability in this context refers to the consistency of results from a fitness test. It means that the test results should be a true reflection of the person's ability. Think about how being motivated or not might affect your fitness test results.

Hint

Fitness testing is normally carried out before you start a training programme, at intervals through the training programme and then again at the end. Think about what should happen to the fitness test scores each time, and how this information could be used.

Hint

Question 3(e) expects two distinct answers, as indicated by the numbering. For each one, you need to give a different reason for fitness testing, and then expand each point to show how each will benefit the participant.

Revision Guide
pages 33 and
34

Hint

In this **assess** question you need to consider both of the test protocols, how you do each test, whether there is anything about the test that makes it difficult to carry out. Look at the strengths and weaknesses of each test in terms of how easy they are to carry out. Finally, you need to come to a conclusion as to which is the most practical for someone to do.

Hint

Practicality is about how easy the fitness test is to complete. Consider factors such as:

- How much the test costs
- Whether the equipment is easy to use
- Whether the equipment is easily available
- How long it takes to complete.

Hint

Your answer must always be in the context of the individual in the scenario, in this case that is James and his weightlifting.

James wants to measure his body composition. Two tests to measure body composition are: bioelectrical impedance analysis (BIA) and waist to hip ratio.

(f) Assess the practicality of **each** of these tests for James.

....

....

....

....

....

....

....

....

....

....

....

6 marks

Total for Question 3 = 16 marks

> Tahlia trains in different types of facilities to increase her fitness for volleyball.

4 (a) Name the **type** of facilities being described:

'The facilities tend to be high quality, but expensive.'

....

....

1 mark

> Tahlia carries out plyometric training to improve her power. Each training session is one hour long. She uses a 4 kg medicine ball during the plyometric drills.

(b) Complete **Table 5** by stating:

(i) the name of the FITT principle represented by each letter

(ii) **one** example of how each principle has been applied to Tahlia's training.

FITT principle	(i) Name	(ii) Example
I	....	....
T	....	....

Table 5

4 marks

Revision Guide
pages 2 and 55

Hint

Remember that there are three different types of providers of fitness training provision:
* public provision
* private provision
* voluntary provision.

Hint

Here you need to complete the table by stating the name of each FITT principle and giving an example. In your example, demonstrate you understand the term by giving key features. For example, if asked to give an example of how continuous training could be applied, mention that the runner should maintain a steady pace at moderate intensity for at least 30 minutes.

Hint

Make sure your examples are linked to the scenario in the question. Here, the example must be applied to Thalia's training in plyometrics.

Revision Guide
page 41

Hint

Think about the differences between the two types of test. Why might the vertical jump test be a better choice for a volleyball player?

LEARN IT!

In the standing broad jump you stand two feet together with your toes up to a line on the ground. Jump forward using two feet and measure the distance travelled from the starting line.

Hint

Question 4d asks you to describe the process that should be followed to complete this test. You need to give enough detail so that the person reading gets a good understanding of how to do the test. Try to make three linked points they would need to do in the order they should do them.

Tahlia tests her progress using the standing broad jump test.

(c) Explain **one** reason why a more valid test might be the vertical jump test.

....

....

....

....

2 marks

(d) Describe how the vertical jump test is carried out.

....

....

....

....

....

....

3 marks

Tahlia designs a training programme to help improve her fitness.

(e) Explain why the following personal information should be used to aid her programme design.

Physical activity history

....

....

....

....

Aims for her sport

....

....

....

....

4 marks

Tahlia includes plyometrics sessions in her training programme.

(f) Explain **one** advantage of plyometric training.

....

....

....

....

2 marks

Total for Question 4 = 16 marks

Revision Guide
page 60

Watch out!

An **aim** is what you want to get out of training, what you want to achieve by the end of the session. An **objective** is how you plan to achieve your aims, e.g., the amount or type of training you need to do. Make sure that you are clear about the differences between these terms.

Hint

Specific personal information should be used when planning a training programme for someone. This includes the person's:

- aims
- objectives
- lifestyle and physical activity history
- attitudes to training.

LEARN IT!

Plyometrics is an explosive type of training that is used to improve power in the part of the body being trained. You can do things like burpees, clapping press-ups, tuck jumps or box jumps.

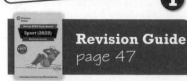

Revision Guide
page 47

 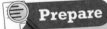
> Jenna is a swimmer who trains regularly with her swimming club. She does well on short-distance races but gets tired during long distance races, often finishing last.

5 Evaluate the use of interval training to improve Jenna's aerobic endurance for swimming.

....

....

....

....

....

....

....

....

....

....

....

6 marks

Total for Question 5 = 6 marks

TOTAL FOR PAPER = 60 MARKS

Practice assessment 2

Answer ALL questions.
Write your answers in the spaces provided.

Some questions must be answered with a cross in a box ☒. If you change your mind about an answer, put a line through the box ☒ and then mark your new answer with a cross ☒.

Revision Guide
pages 32 and 49

Sophia is a rock climber. She needs high levels of muscular endurance for her sport.

1 (a) Which **one** of these statements best describes muscular endurance?

☐ **A** The ability to use voluntary muscles repeatedly over time without them getting tired

☐ **B** The maximum force that can be generated by a muscle or group of muscles

☐ **C** The ability to lift a heavy weight quickly

☐ **D** The ability to perform strength exercises without fatigue

1 mark

Sophia is internally motivated to maintain her training programme as she thinks training is fun.

(b) Name the type of motivation that comes from within the participant.

....

....

1 mark

Sophia tests her body composition using the BMI test.

(c) Which **one** of the following is the unit of measurement for BMI?

☐ **A** mg/m^2

☐ **B** kg/cm^2

☐ **C** kg/m^2

☐ **D** g/cm^2

1 mark

Hint

For Question 1(a), pick the correct answer from the choices offered. Eliminate the ones you know are wrong, then guess if you are still unsure.

Hint

Think about the sport of rock climbing when you are looking at the options. Most rock climbers will spend over 30 minutes completing a climb.

Hint

The key word **name** requires you to recall a piece of information and state it clearly, using the correct terminology.

Hint

Use the number of marks available as a guide to how much you need to include in your answer. This question is worth one mark so does not require a long response.

Hint

Read the options carefully; think about how you carry out the test, and the two things you need to measure.

Hint

Complete means that you need to fill in the empty spaces in the table. For Question 1d(i) you just need to state the type of provision. Then for 1d(ii) explain a disadvantage of this type of provision. The disadvantage should be specific to Sophia (the performer).

Hint

Look for the key information in the descriptions in the first column of the table, for example, the first description mentions expense but also high-quality facilities.

Watch out!

You are given one example questionnaire in the question; don't repeat this in your answer.

Hint

For this **Explain** question, you need to clearly state a reason why Sophia should use a timed-plank test (what it measures) and then give further details to explain why this is relevant to Sophia when rock climbing (how this component of fitness is used in rock climbing).

Sophia wants to make sure she joins a good gym to complete her training, so she looks at the provision available.

(d) Complete **Table 1** by stating:

    (i) the **type** of provision being described

    (ii) **one disadvantage** of the type of provision for the performer.

Description	(i) Type of provision	(ii) Disadvantage of type of provision
Expensive membership costs to allow high standard of facilities with an aim to make a profit.	....	....
Funded by money from local authorities with an aim to make sport accessible to all.	....	....

Table 1

4 marks

Personal information, such as information from a lifestyle questionnaire, should be used when planning a fitness programme.

(e) Name **one** other type of questionnaire Sophia should complete before planning her fitness programme.

....

....

1 mark

Before starting her training programme Sophia takes part in some fitness tests.

(f) Explain **one** reason why Sophia would use a timed plank test to assess her fitness for rock climbing.

....

....

....

....

2 marks

Total for Question 1 = 10 marks

Samuel is a footballer. He tests his fitness regularly. Each picture (**A** and **B**) shows a type of fitness test method.

2 (a) Identify the fitness test method shown in pictures **A** and **B**.

Draw a straight line to match each picture to the correct fitness test method.

Picture

A

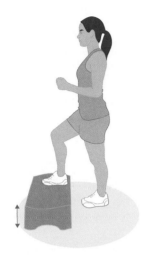

B

Start

Finish

5 metres

10 metres

3.3 m

3.3 m

3.3 m

Fitness test method

T Test

Multi-stage fitness test

Illinois agility run test

Margaria-Kalamen power test

Harvard step test

2 marks

Revision Guide
pages 20, 21, 35, 36 and 43

Hint

Identify means you need to select information from the options given. In this case, it is a list of fitness testing methods.

Hint

The first image (**A**) shows a performer stepping onto a bench. Look at the possible options to see if there is a possible clue in any of the fitness test names.

Hint

Try to use the available information given in the question. For example, in image (**B**) the arrows indicate several changes of direction. Think about the component of fitness being tested when there is a change in direction.

Watch out!

Fitness test methods and fitness training methods are not the same thing. Fitness testing measures our fitness whereas fitness training is used to improve our fitness. Make sure you are clear on the difference.

Revision Guide
pages 13 and 14

Hint

For Question 2(b) you need to know the component of fitness being tested (look back at Question 2(a)) and use this information to start to answer the question. So, identify the component then add further detail to explain why this would improve Samuel's performance in football.

Hint

When **describing**, make sure you give a clear step-by-step account of how to complete the process, in this case the steps you would follow to calculate the aerobic training zone for a 17-year-old.

Hint

The command word **give** requires you to be clear and concise.

Hint

Think about the different technology available, for example, apps for a phone or tablet or heart rate monitors that are worn under clothing.

(b) Explain **one** reason why the component of fitness tested in method **B** would improve Samuel's football performance.

....

....

....

....

2 marks

> Samuel is 17 years old. During part of a training session Samuel will work within his aerobic training zone.

(c) Describe how Samuel would work out his aerobic training zone.

....

....

....

....

....

....

3 marks

> Samuel uses a smart watch to make sure he is training at the correct intensity.

(d) Give **one** advantage to Samuel of using this type of technology during his training.

....

....

1 mark

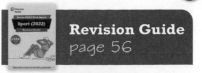

Samuel's training causes adaptations to his cardiovascular and respiratory systems. These adaptations increase his aerobic endurance.

(e) Complete **Table 2** by stating:

   (i) **one** adaptation to each body system as a result of aerobic endurance training

   (ii) why this adaptation will improve Samuel's aerobic endurance.

Body system	(i) Adaptation to body system	(ii) Why this adaptation increases aerobic endurance
Cardiovascular	....	....
Respiratory	....	....

Table 2

4 marks

Total for Question 2 = 12 marks

LEARN IT!

The cardiovascular system is made up of the heart, blood and blood vessels.

LEARN IT!

The respiratory system is responsible for getting air containing oxygen into the body and expelling waste gases such as carbon dioxide.

Hint

Think about how the heart adapts so that it can circulate more blood during exercise.

Hint

Blood transports oxygen, carbon dioxide and nutrients. Think about how an increase in transportation of these could help during exercise.

Watch out!

The role of the cardiovascular system and respiratory system is different, but they are dependent on each other. The respiratory system brings air into the body, the cardiovascular system transports it around the body. Make sure that you are clear about the differences between these body systems.

Revision Guide
pages 19 and 20

Marko plays badminton. He tests his fitness but is concerned his results may not be reliable.

3 (a) Which **one** of the following is a correct definition for reliability of fitness test results?

☐ **A** How accurate a test is so that it measures what it should measure.

☐ **B** How easy a test is to administer.

☐ **C** A test that does not need repeating.

☐ **D** A test that gives consistency of results.

1 mark

(b) State **one** fitness test that can be used to measure reaction time.

....

....

1 mark

Marko completes the Yo-Yo test to measure his aerobic endurance.

(c) Explain **one** reason why the Yo-Yo test would be a more valid test for Marko than the multi-stage fitness test.

....

....

....

....

2 marks

(d) Explain **one** reason why it is important for participants to complete an informed consent form before taking part in fitness testing.

....

....

....

....

2 marks

Marko warms up before every training session.

(e) Explain **two** reasons for warming up before a training session.

1 ....

....

....

....

2 ....

....

....

....

4 marks

Revision Guide
pages 16, 45 and 60

Hint

Make sure you clearly identify one reason for completing an informed consent and then use words such as 'because' to help make sure you are explaining your point.

LEARN IT!

An informed consent form gives information about the test and any risks associated with completing the test. The form is completed when the person taking part signs the form.

Hint

For Question 3(e) you need to give two different answers. Make sure you can think of two separate reasons and give a different expansion for each.

Hint

Don't worry if you don't need to use all available writing space. There should be more than enough room for each response on the assessment.

Revision Guide
page 1

Hint

For this **assess** question you need to consider both components of fitness and explain the pros and cons logically. These must be specific to the context (badminton). Finally, you need to make a judgement about whether the components are important to the badminton player.

Hint

Coordination is needed in any activity that requires the movement of two or more body parts. Think about a game of badminton and:

- when the player needs to move two or more body parts at the same time
- what coordination will allow the badminton player to do
- then think about why this might be important in a game.

Hint

Use a PEEL structure for each component of fitness: **P**oint – make one point; **E**xplain – explain the point; **E**vidence – justify and give evidence for your point and explanation; **L**ink – link back to the question.

LEARN IT!

Power is speed × strength.

Picture C shows Marko about to play a badminton shot.

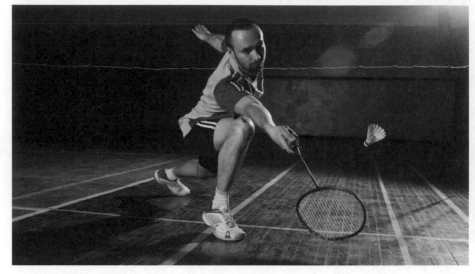

Picture C

Marko has high levels of coordination and power.

(f) Assess the importance of high levels of **coordination** and **power** when playing a game of badminton.

....

....

....

....

....

....

....

....

....

....

....

....

6 marks

Total for Question 3 = 16 marks

Owen is a boxer. He wants to start training to improve his fitness.

4 (a) Name the additional principle of training being described:
        'in order to progress training needs to be demanding enough to
        cause the body to adapt, improving performance'.

....

....

1 mark

Owen joins a boxing club. In the first training session, he
completes a number of fitness tests. The test results show that his
aerobic endurance and agility are both poor.

(b) Complete **Table 3** by stating:

   (i)   a training method that could be used to improve each
         component of fitness

   (ii) how to carry out each of the training methods chosen.

Component of fitness	(i) Training method	(ii) How to carry out the training method
Aerobic endurance	....	....
Agility	....	....

Table 3

4 marks

Revision Guide
pages 47 and 52

Watch out!

There are two groups of principles of training: the basic principles of training (FITT) and the additional principles of training. Make sure you are clear which principles belong to which group.

LEARN IT!

Aerobic endurance training improves the ability of the cardiorespiratory system to transport oxygen and nutrients to the working muscles so the body can work for longer.

Hint

Agility requires quick changes of direction. Think of a training method that uses this type of movement.

Hint

In column (i), you need to briefly state the main features of each training method. You do not go into a lot of detail in column (i).

Revision Guide
page 20

Hint

In a two-mark explain question, there should be two parts to your response, for example, why the test is appropriate and the explanation that links this back to the boxer in the question.

Hint

Think about the component of fitness tested by the multi-stage fitness test and then the relevance of this component of fitness to a boxer.

Watch out!

Be careful when you see the words multi-stage; this is to do with the stages a runner progresses through during the test.

Hint

Think about the main stages of the multi-stage fitness test protocol. For example, think about:

• how the test starts
• the use of equipment in the test
• how far you run
• what happens to the beep sound during the test
• when the test ends.

(c) Explain **one** reason why the multi-stage fitness test would be an appropriate fitness test for Owen.

....

....

....

....

2 marks

Owen tests his fitness using the multi-stage fitness test.

(d) Describe how the multi-stage fitness test is carried out.

....

....

....

....

....

....

3 marks

The boxing club has a few 1 kg, 2 kg and 5 kg free weights that Owen can use in his training.

(e) Explain **one** advantage and **one** disadvantage to Owen of using free weights as part of his training.

Advantage

....

....

....

....

Disadvantage

....

....

....

....

4 marks

Table 4 shows some of Owen's fitness test results.

Fitness test	Rating
One-minute press-up	Average
One minute sit-up	Average
Shoulder flexibility test	Excellent
Grip dynamometer	Poor

Table 4

(f) Explain, using the data in Table 4, **one** component of fitness Owen should train to improve his fitness for boxing.

....

....

....

....

2 marks

Total for Question 4 = 16 marks

Revision Guide
pages 49 and 50

LEARN IT!

Free weights can be used to improve muscular endurance or muscular strength by altering the number of repetitions and the load.

Hint

Read the question carefully to ensure that your answer has the right focus. Question 4e asks for one advantage and one disadvantage, so you need to clearly state the advantage or disadvantage and then provide a reason using a connective word to help you.

Hint

Make use of the additional information given in the question. Think about whether it matters to Owen if there are only a few weights to use or if the weights are relatively light.

Hint

Look for the lowest rating and then consider whether this component of fitness would be important to Owen in his sport.

Revision Guide
page 60

Monica is a long-distance runner. **Table 5** shows Monica's partially completed fitness programme.

Personal information			
Exercise availability:	**Health screening questionnaire results:**	**Activity dislikes:**	**Activity likes:**
Mon-Fri: after 6 p.m. Sunday: Any time.	Asthma	Continuous training on roads	Any other training
Aim: To reduce her marathon time by 10 minutes.			
Objective: To take part in four fartlek training sessions a week.			
Components of fitness: Aerobic endurance			

Table 5

A fitness programme requires a set structure to ensure it is effective in achieving the aim of the participant.

5 Evaluate the use of personal information in designing a suitable fitness training programme for Monica.

....

....

....

....

....

....

....

....

....

....

....

....

....

....

6 marks

Total for Question 5 = 6 marks

TOTAL FOR PAPER = 60 MARKS

Practice assessment 3

Answer ALL questions.
Write your answers in the spaces provided.

Some questions must be answered with a cross in a box ☒. If you change your mind about an answer, put a line through the box ☒ and then mark your new answer with a cross ☒.

Tyler takes part in a fitness test to measure his reaction time.

1 (a) Which **one** of the following tests would Tyler use to measure his reaction time?

☐ **A** 30-metre flying sprint test

☐ **B** Alternate-hand wall-toss test

☐ **C** Ruler drop test

☐ **D** Yo-Yo test

1 mark

(b) Name **one** other reaction time test.

....

....

1 mark

(c) Which **one** of the following is a reason for fitness testing?

☐ **A** Can cause adaptations to body systems

☐ **B** Can improve fitness

☐ **C** Can provide goal setting aims

☐ **D** Can be used as a warm-up

1 mark

Revision Guide
pages 15, 20, 29, 39 and 44

Pearson BTEC Tech Award
Sport (2022)
Revision Guide
FREE

Hint

Mark the box clearly with an X so that the examiner is sure which answer you have chosen. If the examiner is unsure, they will not be able to mark your work as correct.

LEARN IT!

Reaction time is the time taken to respond to a stimulus.

Hint

All of the fitness tests will require some level of reaction time, but only one is specifically designed to test your ability to respond to a stimulus.

Hint

You are asked to **name** another type of reaction time test, so do not repeat any tests already stated in the options in Question 1(a).

Hint

Fitness testing allows us to collect data about our current level of fitness. Think about how this type of data can be used by the performer.

Hint

If asked to **state**, recall the correct name from the specification. For example, one training method to improve **aerobic endurance** would be 'circuit training'.

Hint

In column (ii), give a clear advantage of him needing each component of fitness. For example, if the component of fitness was power, an advantage of working on this would be that he could hit and kick the ball with more force so the ball cleared the goal.

Hint

Look at the information in the question to see which goals could be attained in about a week.

LEARN IT!

A long-term goal is something we want to achieve in the future: a long-term aim.

Hint

In a two-mark **explain** question, there should be two parts to your response. Here this is the reason for setting long-term goals, and the expansion – why this would benefit Tyler.

Tyler plays in goal for his local hockey team. He uses two different training methods to improve his flexibility and agility.

(d) Complete **Table 1** by stating:

(i) **one** method of training to improve each component of fitness

(ii) **one** advantage of training each component of fitness for Tyler's hockey performance.

Component of fitness	(i) Method of training	(ii) Advantage of training this component of fitness
Flexibility		
Agility		

Table 1

4 marks

Tyler motivates himself to improve his fitness by setting long-term goals.

(e) Name **one** other type of goal Tyler should set to give him weekly targets to achieve.

....

....

1 mark

(f) Explain **one** reason why Tyler should set long-term goals.

....

....

....

....

2 marks

Total for Question 1 = 10 marks

Grace is training to improve her performance in netball. She uses two different fitness training methods.

2 (a) Identify the fitness test method shown in pictures **A** and **B**.

Draw a straight line to match each picture to the correct fitness training method.

Picture

A

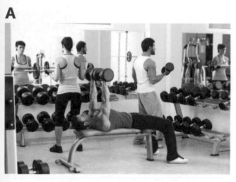

B

Fitness training method

Circuit training

Fartlek training

Free weights

Plyometrics

Static active

2 marks

Revision Guide
pages 45, 47, 49 and 53

Hint

Identify means that you need to choose the correct answer using the information you are given in the pictures. Look at the equipment that is being used. Think about the training methods that would use this type of equipment.

Hint

Have a go at matching the pictures to the training, even if you are not sure. Discount those you know are definitely incorrect. For example, static active is a type of flexibility training, so check if the pictures show this type of training.

LEARN IT!

Fartlek training is where you vary the intensity at which you work in the training session and possibly the terrain.

LEARN IT!

Fitness training methods are used to develop specific components of fitness. You should choose the method once you know the component of fitness you want to improve.

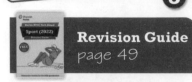

Revision Guide
page 49

LEARN IT!

Muscular endurance is used in events or sports lasting more than 30 minutes. It means that the muscles can contract repeatedly without needing to rest and recover.

Hint

When answering questions where the command verb is **describe** you need to give a clear, account in your own words about how to do something, in this case how to measure muscular endurance.

Hint

Think of the fitness tests you know, and whether any make you work the same set of muscles for a period of time without any rest.

Hint

Be careful not to confuse the basic principles of training, FITT, with the additional principles of training. You need to name an **additional** principle of training.

LEARN IT!

There are seven additional principles of training.

(b) Explain **one** reason why Grace's muscular endurance would improve with regular participation in fitness training method **B**.

....

....

....

....

2 marks

> To make sure her training is effective, Grace measures her muscular endurance.

(c) Describe **one** fitness test method Grace could use to measure her muscular endurance.

....

....

....

....

....

....

3 marks

> Grace applies the principles of training to her fitness programme, making sure the training meets her needs.

(d) Give the additional principle of training that means training should meet the needs of an individual.

....

....

1 mark

Grace has identified she needs to improve her shooting as she misses at least 50% of her shots. She sets herself SMARTER personal goals to address this area of her performance.

(e) Complete **Table 2** by stating:

(i) the name of the SMARTER personal goal represented by each letter

(ii) **one** example of this type of goal that Grace should set to improve her shooting performance.

SMARTER goal	(i) Name of the SMARTER personal goal represented by each letter	(ii) Example of this type of goal
S	....	....
T	....	....

Table 2

4 marks

Total for Question 2 = 12 marks

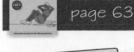

Revision Guide
page 63

LEARN IT!

Goal setting provides direction for behaviour and helps us maintain our focus on the task at hand.

Hint

Use your own experience to help you answer this question. Think about your own training goals and whether any of these would be good examples to use here.

Hint

In Question 2(e) ii make sure your example uses the additional information you are given in the question. Your examples should have something to do with her % shooting success.

Hint

Even if you are not sure of all the answers, complete as much of the table as possible as you will gain marks for any correct answers. For example, if you know one of the SMARTER personal goals, add it to the table even if you have to leave the rest blank.

Hint

Read the question carefully; all of the components of fitness are useful to some of the activities given in the question, but you have been asked which component is important in **all** cases.

Hint

Go through the list of options and for each one, check its importance to all of the events. For example, reaction time is vital to the 100 m sprint, but reflect on whether a quick reaction is required for the throwing events.

Hint

Golfers need to be able to swing the club to hit the ball. The bigger the swing, the greater potential the ball has to travel a long way.

Hint

When Ruby plays golf, it normally takes her 4 hours to complete the course.

Ruby represents her school in shot put, javelin and the 100 m sprint. Ruby also plays golf out of school.

3 (a) Which **one** of the following components of fitness is important to Ruby in **all** of her activities?

☐ **A** Aerobic endurance

☐ **B** Coordination

☐ **C** Muscular endurance

☐ **D** Reaction time

1 mark

(b) State **one** reason why Ruby will need a good level of flexibility to play golf well.

....

....

1 mark

(c) Explain **one** reason why Ruby would also need good aerobic endurance to play golf.

....

....

....

....

2 marks

Ruby regularly tests her fitness.

(d) Explain **one** reason why it is important that Ruby always completes her fitness tests in a consistent testing environment.

....

....

....

....

2 marks

Ruby carries out pre-test procedures before each fitness test.

(e) Explain **two** pre-test procedures that Ruby should carry out before testing.

1 ....

....

....

....

2 ....

....

....

....

4 marks

Revision Guide
pages 16, 17
and 19

Hint

The testing environment is where you take the test; this could be in the gym, on the school field or even in the classroom.

Hint

As well as being where you take the test, the environment refers to the conditions of that environment at the time. Remember these should be consistent. For example, although you may always use the school field for the 12-minute Cooper run, think what might happen to the distance you can achieve if the first time it was a mild, pleasant, dry day and the second time it was heavy rain, muddy and windy.

Hint

When you **explain** for this question, you must give two distinct answers. Make each point by identifying a pre-test procedure and then expand each point to show why this is important.

Revision Guide
page 19

Hint

In this **assess** question, you should give careful consideration to both the reliability and validity of each of the test protocols, then make a judgement about which of these tests, if any, has the better validity or reliability.

Hint

Reliability is about consistency of results. Factors such as the following should all be considered:

- motivation
- calibration of equipment
- compliance with the standardised test procedure.

Hint

Validity is about whether the test actually tests what it is meant to test. These are all recognised tests of aerobic endurance so the tests' results should be similar, but they are not. Think about the test protocols, what Ruby needs to do in the test compared to what she needs to do when playing golf.

Ruby trains to improve her aerobic endurance for golf.

She measures her aerobic endurance at the start and end of a six-week training programme.

Table 3 shows Ruby's ratings for each aerobic endurance fitness test.

Fitness test	Rating of Result (Week 1)	Rating of Result (Week 6)
12-minute Cooper swim	Poor	Poor
Harvard step test	Average	Good
Multi-stage fitness test	Above average	Average

Table 3

(f) Assess the reliability and validity of Ruby's aerobic endurance ratings for **each** of these tests.

....

....

....

....

....

....

....

....

....

....

....

....

6 marks

Total for Question 3 = 16 marks

Thomas plays rugby for a local rugby club. The club is run and organised by its members.

4 (a) Name the **type** of provision being provided by the local rugby club.

....

....

Revision Guide
pages 2 and 55

1 mark

LEARN IT!

There are three different types of providers of fitness training provision:
- public provision
- private provision
- voluntary provision.

Thomas does three, 30-minute SAQ training sessions a week to improve his fitness for rugby. He applies the FITT principles to his training.

(b) Complete **Table 4** by stating:

(i) **one** example of how each principle has been applied to Thomas's training

(ii) how each principle could be applied to the programme to increase Thomas's fitness.

FITT principle	(i) Example	(ii) Application to programme
Frequency		
Time		

Table 4

4 marks

Hint

Think about the type of provision where those organising and running the club are probably not paid to do so.

Hint

In Question 4(b)i in your example, use the information provided in the question, that he trains 3 times a week for 30 minutes

Hint

For Question 4(b)ii you need to think about how you could apply each basic principle to increase the player's fitness. Remember that to increase fitness, you need to gradually overload the body so it has to work slightly harder each time.

Revision Guide
page 36

Revision Guide
page 36

Hint

For Question 4(c), think about the T Test protocol and what Thomas will have to do. This should remind you what component of fitness is being tested. Think about whether Thomas uses this component of fitness in this way in a game.

Hint

Question 4(d) asks you to describe how to do something – what you should do to complete the test. You need to give enough detail so that the person reading your answer gets a good understanding of how to do the test. Try to bring out the key points they would need to do in the order they should do them.

LEARN IT!

The test protocol is the method used to complete the test. Test protocols are standardised so that everyone does them in the same way.

Thomas uses the T Test to measure his progress.

(c) Explain **one** reason why the T Test is a valid test to measure Thomas's rugby fitness.

....

....

....

....

2 marks

(d) Describe the test protocol for the T Test.

....

....

....

....

....

....

3 marks

Thomas designs a new training programme to help improve his fitness.

(e) Explain why the following personal information should be used to aid his programme design.

Objectives

....

....

....

....

Attitude towards training

....

....

....

....

4 marks

The picture shows Thomas taking part in resistance drills as part of his training.

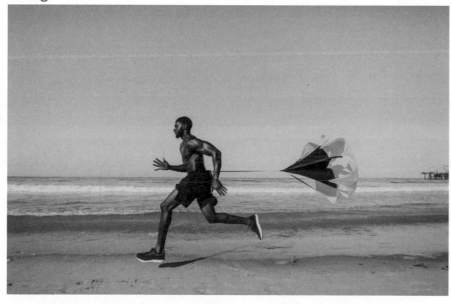

(f) Explain **one** advantage of resistance drills training.

....

....

....

....

2 marks

Total for Question 4 = 16 marks

Revision Guide
pages 51 and 60

Watch out!

An objective is how you plan to achieve your aims. An aim is what you want to get out of training. You need to know the differences between these terms.

Hint

Think how your attitude to training may affect your programme in terms of the activities you do and how hard and often you are willing to work.

Hint

Resistance drills can include hill runs, resistance bands, sleds, parachutes or bungee ropes.

Revision Guide
page 48

Hint

When you **evaluate**, you consider various aspects of a subject's qualities in relation to its context, such as advantages and disadvantages. You need to come to a judgement supported by evidence, which will often be in the form of a conclusion.

Watch out!

Relate your answer to the sport in the question, so that your evaluation is relevant to the question context.

Hint

Begin your answer with a brief description of the two training methods and then evaluate some advantages and disadvantages for how effectively each could improve flexibility and sprint hurdling. Make sure you conclude by making a judgement about which should be used and why.

Hint

Facilitation means to help. This might be one way of remembering that to complete PNF stretching requires the help of another person.

Kenji is a sprint hurdler. He wants to improve his time in the 110 m hurdles but to do so he needs to improve his flexibility.

5 Evaluate which **one** of these training methods Kenji should use to improve his flexibility for sprint hurdling.

- Static stretching
- Proprioceptive neuromuscular facilitation (PNF)

....

....

....

....

....

....

....

....

....

....

....

....

6 marks

Total for Question 5 = 6 marks

TOTAL FOR PAPER = 60 MARKS

Practice assessment 4

Answer ALL questions.
Write your answers in the spaces provided.

Some questions must be answered with a cross in a box ☒. If you change your mind about an answer, put a line through the box ☒ and then mark your new answer with a cross ☒.

Max plays table tennis. He needs quick reactions for his sport.

1 (a) Which **one** of the following components of fitness is required in sports where quick decisions are needed?

☐ **A** Aerobic endurance

☐ **B** Body composition

☐ **C** Muscular endurance

☐ **D** Reaction time

1 mark

Max calculates his 1RM.

(b) Name the component of fitness Max is testing by his 1RM.

....

....

1 mark

During a training session, Max rates his training intensity as 15 using the Borg (6–20) Rating of Perceived Exertion Scale.

(c) Which **one** of the following heart rate values would Max expect to have if he scores 15 on the RPE scale?

☐ **A** 50

☐ **B** 100

☐ **C** 150

☐ **D** 200

1 mark

Revision Guide
pages 1, 4 and 31

Hint

All the components of fitness listed here are important in different sports. To help you select the correct option, you are given key information in the question: 'component of fitness [...] where quick decisions are needed'.

Hint

1RM is an abbreviation used for a common way of testing a component of fitness. The '1' is written as a number for a reason. As this question just asks you to **name**, your answer should be brief.

LEARN IT!

There is a relationship between Rating of Perceived Exertion and heart rate. Make sure you know this relationship: RPE × 10 = HR (bpm).

Hint

Use the relationship between RPE and HR to work out the answer.

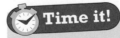 **Time it!**

Don't spend too long on short-answer questions. You need to allow more time to develop your answers for the longer-mark questions.

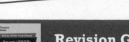

Revision Guide
pages 38, 55
and 60

Hint

Complete means that you need to fill in the empty spaces in the table.

Hint

To complete the first column you need to think of a typical venue for the table tennis club or this type of provision. For example, a typical venue for a public provision table tennis club would be a local authority sports hall.

There is private provision and voluntary provision for table tennis where Max lives.

(d) Complete **Table 1** by stating:

  (i) **one** example of each type of provision

  (ii) **one** advantage of each type of provision.

Provision	(i) Example	(ii) Advantage
Private		
Voluntary		

Table 1

4 marks

Watch out!

You are given one example in the question, so don't repeat this in your answer.

Before taking part in fitness testing, Max completes an informed consent form and a questionnaire.

(e) Name **one** type of questionnaire Max should complete before taking part in fitness testing.

....

....

1 mark

Hint

For this **Explain** question, you need to identify the reason and then give an explanation as to why this is.

Hint

There are other tests of balance Max could have used; think about why this test is more relevant to his sport than the stork stand test. This should help you decide why it is a good test for Max.

Before starting his training programme, Max takes part in some fitness tests.

(f) Explain **one** reason why Max would use the Y balance test to assess his fitness for table tennis.

....

....

....

....

2 marks

Total for Question 1 = 10 marks

Revision Guide
pages 1, 24, 26, 27, 30 and 31

Gareth is a gymnast. He tests his fitness regularly. Each picture (**A** and **B**) shows a type of fitness test method.

2 (a) Identify the fitness test method from the equipment shown in pictures **A** and **B**.

Draw a straight line to match each picture to the correct fitness test method.

Picture

A

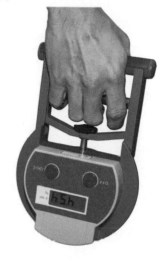

B

Fitness test method

| One minute sit-up test |

| Calf muscle flexibility test |

| Sit and reach test |

| IRM test |

| Grip dynamometer test |

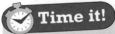
2 marks

Hint

Identify in this case means select your answer from the given list of fitness testing methods.

Hint

The first image (**A**) shows a performer gripping the equipment. Look at the possible options to see if there is a clue in any of the options.

Hint

Before making your choice consider the options and place a mark next to what you think is the correct answer before drawing your line. If you make a mistake, make sure it is clear which line is the error and which line you want to keep.

LEARN IT!

Fitness tests are designed to measure specific components of fitness. For example, the 1RM measures strength.

Time it!

This question is worth 2 marks. You should spend a maximum of 3 minutes on it. Remember to check your answer once you have finished.

Revision Guide
pages 17 and 48

Hint

Calibration of equipment means checking the accuracy of fitness testing equipment before it is used, for example, in the 30 m sprint test stop watches should be set to 0 before starting otherwise the participant will appear to take longer to complete the test than they actually did. Think about how this might apply to Gareth's fitness test.

LEARN IT!

Proprioceptive Neuromuscular Facilitation (PNF) is a technique that is used as a form of flexibility training. Other types of flexibility training include static active stretching and static passive stretching.

Hint

When **describing** make sure you give a clear account of the PNF technique.

LEARN IT!

Fitness tests have set protocols that should be followed to increase consistency of results, giving the test high reliability.

Hint

Give means that you need to give a precise answer that uses correct terminology and language from the specification.

Before carrying out the test shown in **Picture A**, Gareth calibrates the equipment.

(b) Explain **one** reason why calibration of equipment is important for ensuring validity of results.

....

....

....

....

2 marks

Gareth uses Proprioceptive Neuromuscular Facilitation (PNF) technique to work on his flexibility.

(c) Describe Proprioceptive Neuromuscular Facilitation (PNF) technique.

....

....

....

....

....

....

3 marks

Calibration of equipment and level of motivation are two factors that may influence the reliability of a fitness test.

(d) Give **one** other example of a factor that may influence the reliability of a fitness test.

....

....

1 mark

Gareth needs to increase his upper body strength, so takes part in some strength training. To make sure the strength sessions are effective, he applies the additional principles of training to his programme.

(e) Complete **Table 2** by stating:

 (i) the name of the additional principle of training from the description

 (ii) **one** example of how this additional principle could be applied to a strength training programme.

Description	(i) Additional principle of training	(ii) Example applied to strength training
Training should meet the needs of the individual	....	....
Changes to the body due to increased training loads	....	....

Table 2

4 marks

Total for Question 2 = 12 marks

Revision Guide
page 50

Hint

Make sure your answer is clear, for instance, an example of the application of progressive overload would have to show a gradual increase in weight lifted, for example, from 15 kg to 16 kg.

LEARN IT!

Strength training methods use free weights and fixed resistance machines using high loads and low repetitions.

LEARN IT!

The principles of training are classed as basic or additional. The basic principles of training are frequency, intensity, time and type (FITT). The additional principles of training are represented by the letters RIPS VAR, for example, 'R' stands for reversibility.

Watch out!

Make sure you put your answer in the correct space in the table. In this question the example must go in the end column and must link to your answer in the first column, which must link to the description.

Revision Guide
pages 1, 29
and 46

LEARN IT!

A cool down should be performed after every training session. Cooling down returns the body to its pre-exercise state by gradually decreasing the heart rate and breathing rate.

Hint

If you change your mind about your answer, strike through the incorrect response and place a cross in the box for your revised option. Make sure it is clear to the examiner which option you have finally gone for.

Hint

Like **give** and **name** questions, **state** means that you just need to give a clear and concise answer.

Hint

Look for the words in bold, in this case **not**, and make sure your answer only covers this. For example, you know reaction time is needed to make quick decision. So, think about the high jumper and whether they normally need to make quick decisions in their event.

Layla is a high jump athlete. After every training session she always cools down.

3 (a) Which **one** of the following should happen during a cool down?

☐ **A** Gradual increase in heart rate.

☐ **B** Gradual increase in breathing rate.

☐ **C** Carry out a pulse raiser.

☐ **D** Remove lactic acid.

1 mark

Layla regularly tests some components of fitness to see if she is improving.

(b) State **one** reason why Layla does **not** test her reaction time.

....

....

1 mark

Layla needs a fast run up to help her clear the high jump bar.

(c) Explain **one** reason why the 30 m flying sprint test would be a more valid test for games players than a high jump athlete.

....

....

....

....

2 marks

Layla has a clear aim about what she wants to achieve in her sport.

(d) Explain **one** reason why it is important for participants to have a clear aim before planning a fitness programme.

....

....

....

....

2 marks

Layla is training to improve her power.

(e) Explain **two** reasons why the adaptations from power training will improve her high jump performance.

1 ....

....

....

....

2 ....

....

....

....

4 marks

Revision Guide
pages 53, 59, 60 and 61

Hint

When answering questions where the command verb is **explain**, you need to recall a fact, in this case what an aim is, and then provide further details to show why this is important.

Hint

This question expects two distinct answers. Try not to give overlapping answers as each part must be clearly different.

Hint

Adaptations are changes to the body systems as a result of training. If you work your body harder, it adapts so that it finds it easier to cope with the increased workload. Think about the changes to the body due to power training.

Time it!

Look at the mark allocation and divide your time accordingly. This question is worth 4 marks, so you should spend a maximum of 6 minutes on it.

Revision Guide
page 1

Hint

In this **assess** question you should give careful consideration to both components of fitness to judge their relative importance to a high jumper. Is one more important than the other, or are they equally important? You should give clear reasons for your decision.

Hint

Flexibility is needed in any activity that requires a wide range of movement. Think about the picture of the high jumper:

- when they need a wide range of movement
- what this wide range of movement allows the high jumper to do
- then think about why this is important in this event.

Time it!

Make sure you leave enough time to answer the longer questions in your assessment. You need to spend 8 minutes on your answer.

Picture C shows Layla clearing the bar in high jump.

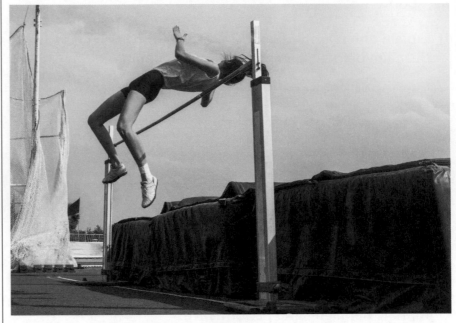

Picture C

Layla has high levels of flexibility and an appropriate body composition for her sport.

(f) Assess the importance of high levels of **flexibility** and an appropriate **body composition** when competing in the high jump.

....

....

....

....

....

....

....

....

....

....

....

....

6 marks

Total for Question 3 = 16 marks

Olivia plays basketball. Due to her fitness training, she develops an increased tolerance to lactic acid.

4 (a) Name **one** type of fitness training that causes an increased tolerance to lactic acid.

....

Revision Guide
pages 47 and 58

1 mark

Hint

The question asks for a type of fitness training. For example, types of fitness training for aerobic endurance would be Fartlek training or circuit training.

Olivia takes part in the fitness training methods of circuit training and plyometrics.

(b) Complete **Table 3** by stating:

  (i) **one** advantage of each fitness training method

  (ii) **one** disadvantage of each fitness training method.

Fitness training method	(i) Advantage of fitness training method	(ii) Disadvantage of fitness training method
Circuit training		
Interval training (for speed)		

Table 3

4 marks

LEARN IT!

Lactic acid builds up when there is insufficient oxygen to break it down. This happens when we work anaerobically (without oxygen), for example, when sprinting.

Hint

Circuit training requires setting up a number of different exercise stations so that participants can work at each station before moving on to a different exercise. Think about how this could be an advantage or disadvantage.

LEARN IT!

Interval training can be used to train aerobic endurance or speed by changing the intensity of the work periods or the length and frequency of the rest periods.

Revision Guide
pages 62 and 63

Olivia is intrinsically motivated and enjoys training. Some of Oliva's friends are only extrinsically motivated.

(c) Explain **one** disadvantage of extrinsic motivation.

....

....

....

....

2 marks

Olivia sets short-term goals to help her achieve her aims.

(d) Describe how Olivia would use time-related, achievable and recorded personal goals when setting a short-term goal.

....

....

....

....

....

....

3 marks

Revision Guide
pages 7 and 11

Olivia is trying to improve her aerobic endurance and speed to improve her basketball performance.

The data in **Table 4** shows the first two weeks and sixth week of Oliva's training programme.

Week	Mon	Tue	Wed	Thur	Fri	Sat	Sun
1	Circuit training 1 hour	Rest day	Fartlek training 1 hour	Interval training 1 hour	Rest day	Basketball match	Rest day
2	Circuit training 1 hour	Rest day	Fartlek training 1 hour	Interval training 1 hour	Rest day	Basketball match	Rest day
6	Circuit training 30 minutes	Rest day	Rest day	Fartlek training 30 minutes	Rest day	Rest day	Rest day

Table 4

(e) Explain, using **Table 4**, how the principles of specificity and reversibility have been applied to the training.

Specificity

....

....

....

....

Reversibility

....

....

....

....

4 marks

Hint

As this is an **Explain** question, make sure you make a point and then expand on it. In this case, say what the principle means and then show where in the training this is applied.

Hint

Make use of the additional information given in the question, you are told she is trying to improve her aerobic endurance and her speed.

Hint

Look at the information provided in the table. You are trying to see how specificity has been applied. Think about the fitness training methods included in the table and the components of fitness they help improve.

Hint

Look for any differences in the training between the weeks. If you find any differences think about what might have happened to cause the training to alter in this way.

LEARN IT!

Specificity means training should match the needs of the sport, or the physical/skill related fitness goal to be developed.

Reversibility means if training stops, or the intensity is lowered, fitness gains from training are lost.

Revision Guide
page 47

Hint

Here you need to state how you would change the circuit and then explain how this will help improve her aerobic endurance.

LEARN IT!

Aerobic endurance is required in events/ sports lasting more than 30 minutes. Aerobic endurance can be improved through:

- continuous training
- Fartlek training
- interval training
- circuit training.

Hint

Make use of the additional information given in the question. Think about the effect on Oliva's aerobic endurance if she changed any one of these parts of her circuit, including the exercises she does at each station

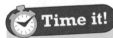 **Time it!**

Review how much time you have spent on the paper so far and check that you've got enough time left to complete the final 6-mark section question.

Olivia completes 6 exercises in her circuit, working for 30 seconds and then resting for 30 seconds. She completes the circuit twice.

Picture D shows some of the stations in Olivia's circuit training session.

Picture D

(f) Explain **one** way Olivia could change her circuit so that her aerobic endurance improves even more.

....

....

....

....

2 marks

Total for Question 4 = 16 marks

Three athletes are training to improve their aerobic endurance. They use the multi-stage fitness test every two weeks to check their progress.

Table 5 shows their fitness test results.

Name	MSFT test 1	MSFT test 2	MSFT test 3
Lin	4.4	5.3	7.1
Richard	5.5	5.6	5.5
Pedro	6.1	6.8	4.5

Table 5

5   Evaluate the effectiveness of each athlete's training using the data in **Table 5**.

....
....
....
....
....
....
....
....
....
....
....
....

6 marks

Total for Question 5 = 6 marks

TOTAL FOR PAPER = 60 MARKS

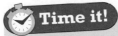

Revision Guide page 15

Hint

Evaluate the effectiveness means that you need to consider how good each person's training was to give them the results they achieved. You need to use the data to come to a justified conclusion as to which had the most effective training programme.

Hint

The higher the score achieved in the multi stage fitness test the better.

Time it!

Before you start writing make a brief plan for longer answers.

Time it!

You need to reserve around 8 minutes to answer the final question and leave yourself a few minutes at the end to check over all your answers.

Time it!

Review how long it took you to complete the assessment. Think about how you could allocate your time differently to improve your performance.

Answers

Use this section to check your answers.

- For questions with clear correct answers, these are provided. If there are alternative correct answers, these are given.
- For questions where answers may be individual or require longer answers, bullet points are provided to indicate key points you could include in your answer, or how your answer could be structured. Your answer should be written using sentences and paragraphs, and might include some of these points but not necessarily all of them.

The questions and sample answers are provided to help you revise content and skills. Ask your tutor or check the Pearson website for the most up-to-date Sample Assessment Material, past papers and mark schemes to get an indication of the actual assessment and what this requires of you. Details of the actual assessment may change so always make sure you are up to date.

Practice assessment 1

(pages 1–12)

1 (a) C – Below average

(b) Flexibility

(c) Calibration of equipment

(d) Individual responses. For example:

Component of fitness	(i) Method of training	(ii) Reason why method of training is suitable
Power	Plyometrics	Plyometrics involves jumping to improve power in the legs, which hurdlers need in order to clear the hurdles.
Speed	Acceleration sprints	This action replicates the start of the hurdle race, sprinting to the first hurdle.

(e) One from:
  - specific
  - achievable
  - realistic
  - time-related
  - exciting
  - recorded.

(f) Individual responses. For example: Raj will be motivated as he gets nearer to his target/sees progress.

2 (a) (i) Frequency

(ii) Aerobic endurance

(b) Individual responses. For example: Fartlek training causes adaptations, for example, capillarisation around the alveoli. This means more oxygen is available to work aerobically.

(c) Individual responses. For example: Ivan gives himself a rating between 6 and 20 depending on how hard he thinks he is working. He then multiplies this number by 10. So, if he rated himself as working hard, his estimated heart rate would be 150.

(d) The internal mechanisms and external stimuli that arouse and direct behaviour.

(e) (i) **From within the performer:** Intrinsic motivation.
  From an external source: Extrinsic motivation.

(ii) **From within the performer:** Individual responses. For example, one from:
  - self-satisfaction/pride in doing something well
  - feeling of accomplishment
  - desire to be recognised
  - enjoyment
  - trying to beat your personal best.

  From an external source: Individual responses. For example, one from:
  - reward/praise from the coach
  - medals
  - trophies
  - cash prize
  - recognition.

3 (a) C – Power

(b) The more muscular strength James has, the more weight he can lift.

(c) Individual responses. For example: to control the distribution of weight evenly, so that he could remain upright when lifting.

(d) Individual responses. For example, one from:
  - If he is motivated to put the same amount of effort into each test, he will achieve more reliable results.
  - If he is not motivated, he won't try so hard and will get a lower fitness rating.

(e) Individual responses. For example:
  - Fitness testing allows James to monitor his performance, so he can check that his programme is still having the desired effect.
  - He can amend his programme, if he is not improving.
  - When he sees improvement, this will motivate him to continue to train.
  - He can use his results to set new fitness aims.

(f) Individual responses. Your answers should show accurate and detailed knowledge and understanding. Your points should be relevant to the question context and provide a well-developed and logical evaluation leading to a fully supported conclusion.
  Your evaluation could include the following points:
  - Body composition is the percentage of body weight that is fat, muscle and bone.

  Bioelectrical impedance analysis (BIA), for example:
  - BIA is the least practical for James as it requires the use of more expensive machinery.
  - It has pre-test requirements, for example, he must be hydrated and must not have exercised or eaten beforehand.
  - However, it is accurate as it runs an electrical current through the body and makes a calculation. It doesn't have the same possible measuring errors of the other tests.

  Waist to hip ratio, for example:
  - It is practical as it requires little equipment, just a tape measure.
  - It is the least expensive of the tests.
  - The calculation is easy: divide waist measurement by hip measurement.
  - You can compare results to a data table to show if you are overweight.
  - Measurements need to be accurate or results will be invalid.
  - It is not very accurate for shorter people.

Conclusion, for example:
- Waist to hip ratio is probably the most practical for James, assuming he is over 5 feet tall, as it is cheap and easy to administer.

4 (a) Private sector provision

(b) Individual responses. For example:

FITT principle	(i) Name	(ii) Example
I	Intensity	Tahlia is using a 4 kg medicine ball.
T	Type	She is using plyometrics to improve her power, needed to jump high in volleyball.
	Time	Tahlia has one-hour training sessions.

(c) Individual responses. For example, one from:
- Both tests measure power but the VJT measures the use of power upwards, which is useful as she needs to jump in volleyball.
- VJT is more sport-specific, as it measures how high she can jump.

(d) Individual responses. For example: Stand sideways next to a wall, feet flat on the floor, reach up as high as you can and mark the wall; jump up and mark the wall at the top of jump; measure the difference.

(e) Individual responses. For example: **Physical activity history:** this is used to show past activity levels, to ensure training builds on these levels and doesn't start too high or too low. Individual responses. For example: **Aims for her sport:** this can help to provide focus and make sure the programme is designed to meet the aims/can be used to see if the programme is working.

(f) Individual responses. For example: an advantage of plyometric training is that it is not expensive as it only requires limited equipment, so anyone can afford to do it.

5 Individual responses. Your answers should show accurate and detailed knowledge and understanding. Your points should be relevant to the question context and provide a well-developed and logical evaluation leading to a fully supported conclusion. Your evaluation could include the following points:

Features of training method, for example:
- Interval training is repeated sets of higher intensity exercise with lower intensity periods for recovery to allow the performer to work at higher intensity again. To work aerobically Jenna should be working at 60–80% HRM. As Jenna's aerobic endurance improves, she will be able to work for longer intervals with shorter rest or recovery periods.

Advantage of training method, for example:
- The advantage of interval training is that it can be carried out in the swimming pool. Jenna could swim a number of lengths, rest and then repeat.

Disadvantage of training method, for example:
- The main disadvantage of interval training is that Jenna needs access to the pool to carry out this training so can't just train whenever she wants.

Evaluation, for example:
- Although there are advantages and disadvantages, as Jenna trains regularly with her swimming club this will give her easy access to a pool to complete her interval training in. This makes her training sport-specific so this will be a perfect method for her.

Practice assessment 2

(pages 13–24)

1 (a) A – The ability to use voluntary muscles repeatedly over time without them getting tired

(b) intrinsic/intrinsic motivation

(c) C – kg/m²

(d) Individual responses. For example:

Description	(i) Type of provision	(ii) Disadvantage of type of provision
Expensive membership costs to allow high standard of facilities with an aim to make a profit.	Private provision	Sophia may not be able to afford to join.
Funded by money from local authorities with an aim to make sport accessible to all.	Public provision	Sophia won't have use of such good equipment/facilities.

(e) PARQ /physical activity questionnaire

(f) Individual responses. For example: The timed plank test measures muscular endurance; rock climbers need muscular endurance so they can continue to use their muscles throughout the climb.

2 (a) **A** Harvard step test **B** Illinois agility run test.

(b) Individual responses. For example, one from:
- Samuel would be able to dodge more effectively and so would be less likely to be tackled.
- He would be better at man marking because when his opponent dodges, he could turn quickly and stay with them.

(c) Individual responses. For example:
The aerobic training zone is a heart rate between 70% and 80% of your maximum heart rate (MHR). First, Samuel would need to calculate his MHR, which is 220 minus his age (220 – 17 = 203). Then, he would need to work out 70% and 80% of his MHR (203 × 0.7 and 203 × 0.8).

(d) Individual responses. For example, one from:
- It can be worn on the wrist easily.
- It will not restrict his movement during training.
- It is easily accessible compared to other forms of technology.

(e)

Body system	(i) Adaptation to body system	(ii) Why this adaptation increases aerobic endurance
Cardiovascular	Cardiac hypertrophy	More blood will be forced out of the heart per beat, increasing the amount of blood that can be circulated per minute to transport more oxygen.
Respiratory	Capillarisation around the alveoli	There will be increased gas exchange, so levels of CO_2 do not build up as it can be breathed out.

3 (a) D – A test that gives consistency of results

(b) Individual responses. For example, one from:
- ruler drop test
- online reaction time test
- reaction test timer.

(c) Individual responses. For example:
- The MSFT requires you to run non-stop, so is not sport-specific as there are changes of intensity in badminton.

- The Yo-Yo test can contain recovery periods, so the Yo-Yo test is more sport-specific to badminton because you don't run continuously in badminton.

(d) Individual responses. For example, one from:
- It shows that the participant signed to show that they were aware of the risks associated with the activities, therefore if they are injured they cannot sue the coach.
- It tells the participant they can drop out at any point, so if they feel it is too challenging, they know they can stop.

(e) Individual responses. For example, two from:
- Warming up before training gradually increases heart rate, to prepare the body for exercise.
- Warming up acts as a pulse raiser, so that more oxygen is available for muscles to use.
- Mobility exercises in the warm up increase the range of movement at the joint.
- Stretching in the warm up reduces the risk of injury.

(f) Individual responses. Your answers should show accurate and detailed knowledge and understanding. Your points will be relevant to the question context and provide a well-developed and logical assessment, which clearly considers the factors and their relative importance and leads to a supported judgement.
Your assessment could include the following points:

Coordination, for example:
- Coordination is the ability to move two or more body parts together, smoothly and accurately.
- This is useful for badminton as good hand–eye coordination means that Mark will hit the shuttlecock accurately with the racket.
- This means Mark will not miss the shuttlecock and be able to return it over the net to continue the rally.
- He will be able to move his feet to the right position to best receive or hit the shuttlecock.

Power, for example:
- Power is speed × strength.
- This is useful in badminton either to hit the shuttlecock hard to the back of the court or to smash.
- This makes it harder for the opponent to return.
- It also enables Mark to move explosively to get in place to receive a smash.

Evaluation, for example:
- Using both coordination and power together enables Mark to make a successful smash shot as he will hit the shuttlecock accurately with a lot of force to win the rally.
- Coordination is most important as without this, Mark will be unable to hit the shuttlecock and continue the rally even if he were really powerful.

4 (a) Progressive overload

(b) Individual responses. Examples include:

Component of fitness	(i) Training method	(ii) How to carry out the training method
Aerobic endurance	• Continuous training • Fartlek training • Interval training • Circuit training	• Run at steady, moderate intensity for at least 30 minutes. • Run at different speeds over different terrain. • Long work period of medium intensity followed by short rest period. • Use a number of different stations, completed in succession with minimal rest between each station.
Agility	• Speed, Agility and Quickness training (SAQ)	• Drills using equipment such as ladders and cones to move quickly in and out.

(c) Individual responses. For example, one from:
- It measures aerobic endurance, which Owen needs to deliver oxygen to his muscles for energy.
- It is a maximal test and boxers need to work at high intensity.

(d) Individual responses. For example: Place cones 20 metres apart. Use the MSFT recording and then run continuously between the cones, keeping to the timing of the bleep until you are unable to keep up with the bleeps.

(e) Individual responses. For example, one each from these lists:
- **Advantage:**
  - Owen can do a number of different exercises and easily vary the load.
  - He can target the exact muscles he wants to work, for either muscular endurance or muscular strength.
  - Free weights allow him to perform a range of movements through the joints.
- **Disadvantage:**
  - The weights do not appear to be heavy enough for Owen, so they will not cause any adaptations to his strength.
  - Movements can be complicated so the exercises are easy to get wrong, which might cause an injury.

(f) Owen should improve his strength because his grip dynamometer test was poor, and without good strength he won't be able to hit his opponent hard.

5 Individual responses. Your answers should show accurate and thorough/detailed knowledge and understanding. Your points will be relevant to the question context and provide a well-developed and logical evaluation leading to a fully supported conclusion.

Your evaluation could include the following points:

Personal information, for example:
- Monica's exercise availability. This is important so that the programme can be designed around activities she can do when she has the free time to exercise.
- The results of any health screening through questionnaires allows an appropriate baseline for training to be set, so knowing she has asthma is important.
- The types of activities Monica likes to do. She doesn't like to do continuous road running but she is happy with any other training method, so road running shouldn't be used.
- Including the aim means it can be checked to see it is realistic. For example, if she had said she wanted to take an hour off her time, this would probably be too ambitious.
- By including the objective Monica has stated how she intends to meet her aim.

Evaluation, for example:
- Having an appropriate baseline to start the training from is essential; without this the training could be set too high, causing demotivation when not achieved, or even injury.
- Knowing what training she likes and when she can train means the programme can be tailored to this, so Monica is more likely to continue training.
- Without an aim, her objectives cannot be checked to see that the programme will work. An aim is therefore essential.
- You should also consider how the principles of training will be applied in the training so that progress can be made safely.
- Using a range of personal information is essential to make sure that a training programme is suitable in terms of meeting the individual's aim, and making the training enjoyable and therefore sustainable.

Practice assessment 3

(pages 25–36)

1 (a) C – Ruler drop test

(b) Online reaction time test/reaction test timer

(c) C – Can provide goal setting aims

(d) Individual responses. For example:

Component of fitness	(i) Method of training	(ii) Advantage of training this component of fitness
Flexibility	• Static active • Static passive • PNF	• He will be able to stretch further to block a shot at goal. • He will find it easier to stretch to reach shots to corners of goal. • He is less likely to be injured.
Agility	• Speed, Agility and Quickness training (SAQ)	• He will be able to quickly guard the different areas of the goal, for example top left corner to bottom right. • He can change direction quickly to stop the next shot.

(e) Short-term goals

(f) Individual responses. For example, one from:
- His long-term goal gives him something substantial to work towards, which will motivate him as he slowly moves towards his target.
- His long-term goal gives him something difficult to work towards, and this gives direction for short-term goals.
- His long-term goal gives focus for a training plan so training is likely to be more structured/effective.

2 (a) **A** Free weights   **B** Circuit training

(b) Individual responses. For example, one from:
- She will be constantly working her muscles, causing them to adapt to the additional use.
- Several stations will use the same muscles, which causes strain on the muscles, causing them to adapt.
- The training will cause capillarisation around the muscles, increasing oxygen delivery to the muscle.
- The muscle adapts to increase oxygen delivery, so the muscles take longer to fatigue.

(c) Individual responses. For example, one from:
- In the one-minute press-up test, start with your arms and body in a straight position. Continually lower your body so that your shoulders are in line with your elbows, then push back up.
- In the one-minute sit-up test, lie on a mat with knees bent, feet on floor and continually sit-up to 90° position, then return to floor.

- In the timed plank test, lie flat, placing your forearms on the floor under your shoulders. Push into the plank position and time how long you can stay there.

(d) Individual needs

(e)

SMARTER goal	(i) Name of the SMARTER personal goal represented by each letter	(ii) Example of this type of goal
S	Specific	I want to reduce the number of missed shots by 10% To increase shots on target to 60%
T	Time	I want to complete this goal in six weeks.

3 (a) B – Coordination

(b) Individual responses, for example, one from:
- She would be able to hit the golf ball further with good shoulder flexibility.
- She would be able to take a bigger swing and make the ball go further.

(c) Individual responses, for example, one from:
- Golf lasts longer than 30 minutes. If Ruby has poor aerobic endurance, she will become fatigued and not play as well.
- Good aerobic endurance will mean that she can maintain the quality of her play, as her muscles will not get fatigued.

(d) Individual responses:
- Conditions should always be the same, so that it is clear that any differences in results are down to changes in fitness, not the test method.
- This will reduce the number of variables, which could affect her results.

(e) Individual responses, for example, two from:
- She should calibrate any equipment she uses, so that her results are accurate.
- She should complete a PAR-Q, to make sure that she is physically fit to carry out maximal tests such as the MSFT.
- She should complete an informed consent form, so that she knows what is expected of her.
- She should complete a pre-fitness test check, to ensure it is safe for her to exercise.

(f) Individual responses. Your answers should show accurate and detailed knowledge and understanding. Your points should be relevant to the question context and provide a well-developed and logical evaluation leading to a fully supported conclusion.
Your evaluation could include the following points:

Reliability, for example:
- The results should be consistent.
- The results for the 12-minute Cooper swim appear reliable as the same result is achieved both times. However, if the results are reliable, it shows the training is not being effective as you would expect the rating to improve.
- The rating does improve for the Harvard step test; this is inconsistent with the result for the Cooper swim.
- The results for the MSFT get worse.
- The reliability of the tests has been affected; this could be down to the motivation of the performer.
- Alternatively, it could be due to the test being carried out differently each time.

Validity, for example:
- The results should be valid as they are all recognised tests of aerobic endurance, therefore measure what they say they measure.
- The test results have different levels of validity.
- None of the tests exactly mirror the actions carried out by the golfer.
- If Ruby is a poor swimmer, she will find it difficult to progress in the Cooper swim test.
- She does not need to step up and down on a golf course, although at least the Harvard step test is not maximal.
- She does not have to work to exhaustion in golf, unlike in the MSFT.

Evaluation, for example:
- The results are not reliable as the results are not consistent, therefore other factors must have affected the results. For example, Ruby may have been highly motivated the first time she completed the MSFT but not motivated to complete the test a second time, reducing the effort she made and the score she achieved.
- Overall, the results are not valid for a golfer as the three tests all give different ratings. The 12-minute Cooper swim is probably least valid as it relies on the ability of the performer to swim, something which Ruby does not need to do for her sport.
- The most valid and reliable results are probably from the Harvard step test as these do improve, and the test is submaximal and on land.

4 (a) Voluntary

(b) Individual responses, for example:

FITT principle	(i) Example	(ii) Application to programme
Frequency	Trains 3 times per week	Increase the number of times he trains
Time	Each session is 30 minutes	Increase the length of the training session

(c) Individual responses, for example, one from:
- The T Test measures agility, which Thomas needs to dodge defenders.
- Thomas will need to sidestep as quickly as possible during part of the test, which makes it specific to his sport.
- The movements required in the T Test match those in rugby, for example, when Thomas is side-stepping to mislead an opponent.

(d) Individual responses, for example:
Four cones are set out in the shape of a T. When the stopwatch starts, sprint the length of the T from cone 1 to cone 2 (10 m); sidestep to cone 3 (5 m) and then to cone 4 (5 m), and run back down the length of the T to cone 1.

(e) Individual responses, for example one from each of:

Objectives:
- Objectives show how you intend to achieve your aims. Without them, training would be less targeted.
- Objectives show the training and component of fitness, which will be used to achieve the aim.
- If you didn't have objectives, it wouldn't be clear how you would meet your aim, so your training programme might not work.

Attitude towards training:
- Our attitudes affect how hard we are willing to work, so if we know how hard we are likely to work, we can plan a programme that we will stick to.
- Our attitudes affect the activities we want to do, therefore they help when planning training that will be motivating.

(f) Individual responses, for example, one from:
- Resistance drills training makes you work harder, so you should develop speed quicker.
- It increases the force generated, so you should develop quicker acceleration.

5 Individual responses. Your answers should show accurate and detailed knowledge and understanding. Your points should be relevant to the question context and provide a well-developed and logical evaluation leading to a fully supported conclusion. Your evaluation could include the following points:

The basic features of each training method:
- Static stretching can be done independently (static active) or with another person (static passive). The athlete can target a specific muscle or muscle group by stretching a muscle and holding the stretch for over 12 seconds.
- PNF stretching needs the help of another person to hold the stretch while the athlete pushes against them.
- The athlete then relaxes the muscle and the person helping stretches the muscle a little further. This is repeated three times.

Some advantages of each training method, for example:
- One advantage of static stretching is that you can tailor it to any sport, so Kenji could target his hips in particular to make them flexible enough to achieve the low position over the hurdles. Also, you don't need any specialist equipment and can do it on your own, so Kenji wouldn't need to rely on anyone else being available when he wanted to train.
- PNF helps to develop flexibility at a faster rate than any other training method, so Kenji would see better results sooner. It also needs minimal equipment.

Some disadvantages of each training method, for example:
- The main disadvantage of static stretching is that it will be limited in terms of increasing his flexibility. This is because it only uses the regular range of motion for the muscle at the joint.
- A disadvantage of PNF stretching is that the person helping needs to be experienced so that they know how far to stretch the muscle, otherwise they would cause Kenji an injury, meaning that he could not race.

Evaluation, for example:
- While both training methods have advantages and disadvantages, as Kenji needs to increase his flexibility in order to get better he should use PNF, provided he has an experienced person to help him. This way his flexibility will increase faster and his sprint hurdling time will improve.

Practice assessment 4

(pages 37–49)

1 (a) D – Reaction time

(b) Strength

(c) C – 150

(d) Individual responses, for example:

Provision	(ii) Example	(i) Advantage
Private	• Private health club, for example, Virgin Active; David Lloyd • Private golf clubs	• Latest equipment • Modern facilities • Offer specialist facilities/ coaching
Voluntary	• Table tennis club in village hall • Community rugby club	• Affordable for all users as non-profit making • Spread cost as normally weekly subscription

(e) Individual responses, for example, one from:
- PAR-Q
- Lifestyle
- Physical activity history.

(f) Individual responses, for example, one from:
- The Y balance measures dynamic balance, which is important for a table tennis player so they can remain stable to make an accurate shot with good technique, even when moving.
- It is more sport-specific, as he needs to maintain his balance while he is moving.

2 (a) **A** Grip dynamometer test **B** Sit and reach test

(b) Individual responses, for example, one from:
- Calibrating the grip dynamometer ensures the results are accurate, therefore the equipment is measuring what it is supposed to measure.
- Standard data tables are used to rate a person's fitness based on results from a test. If the equipment isn't calibrated, the data tables will give a false rating.
- Training programmes are developed based on fitness test results. If the equipment isn't calibrated, the training programme could be set up incorrectly.

(c) Individual responses, for example:

The muscle is stretched by a partner. The muscle is then contracted isometrically, and held for 10 seconds before relaxing and then repeating. This will inhibit the stretch reflex to improve flexibility.

(d) Individual responses, for example, one from:
- Experience of the person administering the test
- Conditions of the testing environment
- Always running the test in the same conditions
- Always following the standardised test procedure.

(e) Individual responses, for example:

Description	(i) Additional principle of training	(ii) Example applied to strength training
Training should meet the needs of the individual	individual differences	Gareth could add chest press exercises to improve his upper body strength at an appropriate weight for his ability.
Changes to the body due to increased training loads	adaptation	Gareth could lift heavier weights due to hypertrophy.

3 (a) D – Remove lactic acid

(b) Individual responses, for example, one from:
- No need to make quick decisions in high jump.
- You do not have a stimulus to respond to in high jump.
- Layla decides when to start her jump so reaction time is not a factor.

(c) Individual responses, for example, one from:
- Because this test is from a running start, it is like the skills used in a game.
- Games players may be jogging back to defend and then have to sprint, so they are not sprinting from a standing start.
- Although high jumpers need speed in their run-up, it is not a flat-out sprint.
- High jumpers start from a stationary position, whereas games players are likely to be moving already.

(d) Individual responses, for example, one from:
- Having a clear aim provides motivation, because you know what you are trying to achieve.
- It gives a clear idea about what you want to achieve, to give a focus for your training.
- You can record what you want to achieve, which means you can check that your training will lead to this.

(e) Individual responses, for example, any two from:
- Muscle hypertrophy will allow her to generate more force to jump higher.
- Increased tendon strength means she is less likely to tear a tendon during an explosive take-off.
- Increased ligament strength means she is less likely to injure herself so she can carry on training.
- Increased bone density means she is less likely to fracture and be absent for a long time from her sport

(f) Individual responses. Your answers should show accurate and detailed knowledge and understanding. Your points should be relevant to the question context and provide a well-developed and logical evaluation leading to a fully supported conclusion.
Your evaluation could include some of the following points:

Flexibility, for example:
- Flexibility is the range of movement possible at a joint.
- It is useful as it allows the performer to arch the back/ create the required shape.
- This means Layla will develop a better technique and is therefore more likely to clear the bar.

Body composition, for example:
- Body composition is the percentage of body weight that is fat, muscle and bone.
- Too much fat or too much muscle will make the body heavier than it should be.
- However, Layla needs enough muscle to provide power to clear the bar.
- Therefore, she needs correct body composition otherwise she will be too heavy to lift her body over the bar.

Evaluation, for example:
- Using both flexibility and an appropriate body composition together enables Layla to get sufficient height off the floor and the arched body shape to clear higher heights in her event.

4 (a) Individual responses, for example, one from:
- Speed training
- Acceleration sprints
- Speed interval training
- Resistance drills

(b) Individual responses, for example:

Fitness training method	(i) Advantage of fitness training method	(ii) Disadvantage of fitness training method
Circuit training	• The variety of stations can be motivating. • You can create a circuit without equipment. • You can develop aerobic endurance and muscular endurance.	• Needs time to set it up. • Takes time to plan what to do at each station. • Needs to be enough time in the session to explain what you do at each station.
Interval training (for speed)	• Easy to apply progressive overload. • Can be tailored to specific sports. • No special equipment required.	• Can become boring due to repetitions. • Needs careful planning to make sure you are working at correct intensity.

(c) Individual responses, for example, one from:
- If we are extrinsically motivated, we do things for the rewards we gain, so if there are no rewards, we will stop training.
- Extrinsic motivation comes from outside the performer, so if the thing that is extrinsically motivating is removed, the performer will have no drive to carry on with the training.

(d) If her goal is time-related, she will have a deadline to complete the goal by; if it is achievable, it means it has to be something that she will be able to do in the timeframe; and if it is recorded, it means she will make a note of the goal so she doesn't forget it or change it accidentally.

(e) Individual responses, for example:

Specificity
- Acting on the specificity principle means matching training to the requirements of the activity. By including circuit training Olivia can set up a basketball circuit train basketball skills, e.g., shooting; by including Fartlek training, she will be working on her aerobic endurance; by including circuit training, she will be working on her aerobic endurance.

Reversibility
- The principle of reversibility asserts that when a person reduces training, they will lose adaptations/training effects; or when they stop training, they will lose fitness. By week 6 Olivia has increased the number of rest days and decreased the amount of time she trains for.

(f) Individual responses, for example, one from:
- Increase the length of time worked at each station. so she has to work for longer.
- Decrease the amount of rest time, so she has less time to recover between stations.
- Change the stationary passing exercise for a more active one, so she has to work harder for longer.

5 Individual responses. Your answers should show accurate and detailed knowledge and understanding. Your points should be relevant to the question context and provide a well-developed and logical evaluation leading to a fully supported conclusion. Your evaluation could include the following points:

Lin, for example:
- Lin's programme is working.

- She is showing that her aerobic endurance is improving as she is able to reach higher levels on the MSFT every two weeks.
- Therefore, she must be applying progressive overload.

Richard:
- Richard's programme is not working.
- His aerobic endurance is the same in the final session as it was when he started.
- Therefore Richard cannot be applying progressive overload.
- Richard needs to gradually increase the intensity he works at if he wants to improve.

Pedro:
- Pedro's programme is not working.
- The second set of tests show he has improved a lot, but he can't maintain this.
- His aerobic endurance is worse at the end of the programme than when he started.
- Therefore, his results show reversibility, which suggests that he may have been overtraining to show such a big increase which could have then led to injury.

Evaluation, for example:
- Lin has the most effective training programme as she has made consistent progress over the training programme, despite starting the programme with the lowest level of aerobic endurance. She now has greater aerobic endurance than both Richard or Pedro.

Notes

Notes

Notes

Notes